Unmasking the Enemy Within

Understanding Colorectal Cancer and Empowering Prevention

By

Shirley L. Brooks

Table of contents

Introduction

Colorectal disease, a term frequently connected with dread and vulnerability, is an imposing foe that influences a large number of lives around the world. A kind of disease emerges in the colon or rectum, two crucial parts of our stomach-related framework. Sadly, the incidence of colorectal cancer is still on the rise, so we must learn more about the disease and take steps to help prevent it.

Millions of people worldwide are affected by colorectal cancer, a prevalent and potentially fatal disease. With its high death rates, understanding this type of disease and enabling avoidance methodologies are of the most extreme significance. One significant part of battling colorectal disease is early identification and counteraction. Individuals have a better chance of surviving and receiving successful treatment if the disease is detected early. Besides, executing preventive measures can essentially lessen the gamble of creating colorectal disease through and through. In this article, we will dive into the meaning of early discovery and anticipation in understanding colorectal disease, revealing insight into the different procedures and measures that can be taken to alleviate its effect on people and networks.

In this extensive aid, we will dive into the intricacies encompassing colorectal malignant growth, its commonness in the public eye, and the effect it has on people and networks. By acquiring a more profound comprehension of this illness, we can outfit ourselves with information and systems to battle its beginning, further develop early discovery rates, and at last save lives.

All through this investigation, we will investigate the study of disease transmission of colorectal malignant growth, featuring expanding commonness and the elements that add to its turn of events. We will dive into the gamble factors, both hereditary and ecological, revealing insight into the significance of way-of-life decisions in relieving the gamble of this illness. By getting a handle on the meaning of early identification and screening, we will engage ourselves to assume responsibility for our well-being and urge others to do likewise.

Go along with us as we leave on an excursion to grasp colorectal disease, its predominance in the public eye, and the urgent job we as a whole play in counteraction. Together, we can arm ourselves with information, move mindfulness, and work towards a future where the effect of colorectal disease is radically decreased.

Chapter 1: The Hidden Threat

Colorectal malignant growth, frequently alluded to as a secret danger, represents a huge well-being chance for people around the world. While the illness may not generally manifest clear side effects in its beginning phases, it can quickly advance and become dangerous whenever left undetected. Understanding the gamble factors and hereditary inclinations related to colorectal malignant growth is pivotal in distinguishing people who might be at a higher gamble and carrying out preventive measures.

Colorectal cancer is brought on by several risk factors. Age is a critical component, with the illness being more common in people beyond 50 years old. People with a family background of colorectal malignant growth or certain hereditary circumstances, for example, Lynch's condition or familial adenomatous polyposis (FAP), are likewise at an expanded gamble. Other gamble factors incorporate an individual history of fiery gut sickness, like Crohn's illness or ulcerative colitis, a stationary way of life, stoutness, smoking, exorbitant liquor utilization, and an eating routine high in red and handled meats.

Additionally, genetic predispositions play a significant role in the development of colorectal cancer. Certain quality transformations, like changes in the APC, KRAS, and TP53 qualities, have been connected to an expanded gamble of colorectal disease. These genetic predispositions can be passed down from one generation to the next or develop naturally.

Perceiving these gamble factors and hereditary inclinations is vital in distinguishing people who might require more continuous screenings or particular preventive measures. Precancerous polyps or early-stage colorectal cancer can be detected through routine screenings like colonoscopies, which enables prompt intervention and improved treatment outcomes. Moreover, way of life changes, for example, keeping a sound weight, taking part in customary active work, embracing a decent eating regimen rich in organic products, vegetables, and entire grains, and keeping away from tobacco and extreme liquor utilization, can essentially diminish the gamble of creating colorectal disease.

Also, understanding the secret danger of colorectal malignant growth requires a thorough investigation of the gamble factors and hereditary inclinations related to the sickness. By recognizing people who might be at a higher gamble, medical care experts can carry out designated preventive measures and screenings, eventually diminishing the weight of colorectal disease and further developing by and large well-being results.

Colorectal malignant growth, frequently alluded to as a secret danger, represents a critical well-being hazard to people around the world. In its early stages, the disease may not always show obvious symptoms, but it can quickly progress and become life-threatening if left untreated. Investigating the job old enough, family ancestry, and way of life decisions is vital in grasping the secret dangers of colorectal malignant growth and executing powerful preventive measures.

Age plays a critical part in the improvement of colorectal malignant growth. The illness is more common in people beyond 50 years old, with the gamble expanding dramatically as time passes. This stresses the significance of customary screenings, like colonoscopies, as people arrive at this age bunch. Early location through screenings can recognize precancerous polyps or beginning phase colorectal disease, empowering opportune intercession and further developed therapy results.

Family ancestry likewise assumes a significant part in colorectal disease risk. People who have the disease in their family, especially first-degree relatives (parents, siblings, or children), are more likely to get it. This proposes a potential hereditary inclination that builds helplessness to colorectal disease. It is fundamental for people with a family background of the illness to illuminate their medical services suppliers, as they might require more incessant screenings or specific preventive measures.

Way of life decisions is one or more huge figure in the improvement of colorectal malignant growth. Undesirable propensities, like a stationary way of life, corpulence, smoking, and unnecessary liquor utilization, have been connected to an expanded gamble of colorectal disease. The risk of developing the disease can be significantly reduced by engaging in regular physical activity, maintaining a healthy weight, avoiding tobacco, and limiting alcohol consumption. Furthermore, dietary decisions assume an essential part, with eating fewer carbs high in red and handled meats being related to an expanded gamble of colorectal disease. Embracing a fair eating regimen wealthy in organic products, vegetables, entire grains, and incline proteins can assist with moderating this gamble.

Understanding the secret dangers of colorectal malignant growth requires a complete investigation of old enough, family ancestry, and way of life decisions. Individuals can take preventative measures to lower their risk by recognizing the impact of these factors, and healthcare providers can implement specific preventive measures. For individuals with a family history of colorectal cancer, regular screenings, lifestyle modifications, and genetic counseling can significantly contribute to the early detection and prevention of the disease, thereby improving overall health outcomes.

Chapter 2: The Veil of Symptoms

Colorectal disease frequently takes cover behind a cloak of side effects that can undoubtedly be confused with other normal illnesses. Perceiving the normal signs and side effects related to this sickness is essential in early recognition and convenient therapy. By getting and monitoring these pointers, people can look for clinical consideration and possibly get the colorectal disease at a prior stage when treatment results are by and large better.

One of the most well-known side effects of colorectal disease is an adjustment of entrails propensities. This might incorporate steady runs or blockage, or a sensation of fragmented defecations. People may likewise see an adjustment in the consistency of their stool, for example, stools becoming smaller or pencil-slight. Furthermore, the presence of blood in the stool, both dazzling red or dim and delayed, can be a huge admonition sign.

Unexplained weight reduction is another side effect that ought not to be overlooked. If a singular encounters a critical and unexpected weight reduction with no progressions in diet or exercise, it could be a sign of a hidden medical problem, including colorectal disease. Weight loss can also be accompanied by common symptoms like weakness and fatigue.

Relentless stomach uneasiness, like spasms, torment, or bulging, ought to likewise raise concerns. While these side effects can be brought about by different variables, if they endure for a drawn-out period, it is fundamental to counsel a medical care professional to preclude colorectal malignant growth as a likely reason.

At times, colorectal malignant growth can prompt rectal draining or the sensation of inadequate departure after a defecation. These side effects can be disturbing and ought to incite people to immediately look for clinical consideration.

It is vital to take note that not every person with colorectal disease will encounter side effects, particularly in the beginning phases. To this end, ordinary screenings, like colonoscopies, are vital for early location, even without a trace of side effects.

Monitoring these normal signs and side effects of colorectal disease can assist people with perceiving likely advance notice signs and making a proper move. It is significant not to excuse or disregard these side effects, as they might show a fundamental medical problem that requires clinical consideration. By looking for convenient clinical consideration and going through suggested screenings, people can expand their possibilities by identifying colorectal disease early, further developing treatment results, and possibly saving lives.

Importance of recognizing warning signs

The shroud of side effects that can go with colorectal disease frequently camouflages itself as a normal illness, making it barely noticeable or excusing possible admonition signs. For the early detection and treatment of colorectal cancer, however, it is crucial to recognize these symptoms and comprehend their significance.

One of the vital purposes behind perceiving advance notice signs is the potential for early mediation. Colorectal malignant growth, when distinguished in its beginning phases, is bound to be treatable and has higher endurance rates. By being careful and mindful of the side effects, people can look for clinical consideration speedily, permitting medical services experts to direct fitting tests and screenings to affirm or preclude colorectal malignant growth.

In addition, individuals can differentiate between potential red flags and normal bodily changes by recognizing warning signs. Numerous side effects related to colorectal malignant growth, for example, changes in gut propensities, stomach uneasiness, unexplained weight reduction, and rectal dying, can undoubtedly be credited to different elements like dietary changes, stress, or minor stomach-related issues. However, it is essential to see a medical professional to rule out colorectal cancer and ensure proper diagnosis and treatment if these symptoms persist or get worse over time.

One more justification behind perceiving advance notice signs is the possibility of forestalling the movement of the illness. Colorectal malignant growth frequently begins as precancerous polyps, which can be identified and eliminated during routine screenings like colonoscopies. By perceiving side effects and looking for clinical consideration, people can go through vital screenings and preventive measures, diminishing the gamble of polyps forming into disease or recognizing malignant growth at a prior stage when treatment choices are more successful.

In addition, it can be beneficial to one's overall well-being to recognize warning signs. Anxiety and stress can rise as a result of ignoring or dismissing symptoms, which can hurt a person's mental health. By recognizing and tending to side effects expeditiously, people can assume command over their well-being, reduce concerns, and possibly forestall or oversee colorectal disease all the more successfully.

Taking everything into account, perceiving the admonition signs related to colorectal malignant growth is significant for early location, ideal treatment, and avoidance. By being proactive and mindful of changes in entrails propensities, stomach uneasiness, weight reduction, rectal dying, and other likely side effects, people can look for clinical consideration expeditiously, possibly prompting further developed results and a higher opportunity for fruitful treatment. It is fundamental to pay attention to our bodies, pay attention to our gut feelings, and focus on our well-being by perceiving and following up on these advance notice signs.

Chapter 3: Unmasking the Enemy

Exposing the foe with regards to colorectal malignant growth advancement includes understanding the stages through which the sickness advances. Colorectal disease regularly occurs throughout some undefined time frame, beginning as harmless polyps in the colon or rectum that can ultimately change into dangerous developments. Analyzing the phases of colorectal malignant growth improvement can reveal insight into the movement of the sickness and give important experiences to early recognition, counteraction, and therapy.

Stage 0: At this beginning phase, the colorectal disease is restricted to the deepest layer of the colon or rectum and has not yet attacked further layers or spread to local lymph hubs. This stage is often portrayed by the presence of strange cells in the coating of the colon or rectum, which might shape little, noncancerous developments called polyps.

Stage I: Disease at this stage has developed through the deepest layer of the colon or rectum and may have arrived at the center layers of the digestive wall. Be that as it may, it has not spread past the colon or rectum to local lymph hubs or different organs. Early identification and mediation at this stage can be urgent in forestalling further movement of the sickness.

Stage II: The cancer may have invaded nearby tissues and broken through the wall of the colon or rectum at this point, but it has not yet spread to lymph nodes or other organs. The cancer is as yet limited, and therapy choices are many times more successful as of now.

Stage III: At this exceptional stage, the disease has spread to local lymph hubs but has not metastasized to far-off organs. It might have developed through the mass of the colon or rectum and attacked close by tissues, expanding the gamble of spreading to different pieces of the body. Therapy for stage III colorectal malignant growth for the most part includes a blend of a medical procedure, chemotherapy, and radiation treatment.

Stage IV: This is the most progressive phase of colorectal disease, where the malignant growth has metastasized to far-off organs like the liver, lungs, or different pieces of the body. Therapy at this stage centers around overseeing and controlling the spread of malignant growth, as well as giving palliative consideration to work on personal satisfaction.

Exposing the adversary in colorectal disease includes perceiving the potential for movement through these stages and making proactive strides toward early recognition, screening, and preventive measures. Understanding the phases of colorectal malignant growth advancement is significant in bringing issues to light, advancing normal screenings, and supporting for way of life and dietary changes that can diminish the gamble of creating colorectal disease. Individuals and healthcare professionals can collaborate to effectively combat colorectal cancer by shedding light on the disease's progressive nature.

Risk Factors of Colorectal Cancer

A few gamble factors have been related to an improved probability of creating colorectal malignant growth, including:

1. Age: The gamble of colorectal malignant growth increases with age, with most cases happening in people beyond 50 years old.

2. Family ancestry: Having direct relations, like guardians, kin, or youngsters, who have had colorectal malignant growth or specific sorts of polyps can build the gamble of fostering the sickness.

3. Individual history of colorectal disease or polyps: People who have recently had colorectal malignant growth or particular sorts of polyps are at an expanded gamble of fostering the infection once more.

4. Bowel inflammation disorders: Persistent fiery states of the colon, like ulcerative colitis and Crohn's illness, can lift the gamble of creating colorectal disease.

5. Hereditary conditions: Certain hereditary disorders, for example, familial adenomatous polyposis (FAP) and innate nonpolyposis colorectal malignant growth (HNPCC), can incline people toward a higher gamble of colorectal disease.

6. Way of life factors: Colorectal cancer has been linked to poor diet, inactivity, obesity, smoking, excessive alcohol consumption, and a diet high in red and processed meats.

7. Diabetes: People with type 2 diabetes might have a higher gamble of creating colorectal malignant growth.

8. Race and identity: African American people have a higher frequency of colorectal malignant growth contrasted with other racial and ethnic gatherings.

People and healthcare professionals can make better decisions about screenings, lifestyle changes, and preventative measures to lower their risk of developing colorectal cancer if they are aware of these risk factors. Moreover, early discovery and way of life changes can assume a critical part in forestalling or overseeing colorectal malignant growth.

The biology and progression of the disease

Colorectal malignant growth, in the same way as other different kinds of disease, occurs because of hereditary transformations and adjustments in the typical science of the cells in the colon or rectum. The sickness regularly advances through a few phases, beginning with the development of harmless polyps that can ultimately change into carcinogenic developments. Understanding the science and movement of colorectal disease is fundamental to creating successful anticipation systems, demonstrative methods, and treatment choices.

The movement of colorectal disease includes a progression of hereditary changes and modifications that add to the uncontrolled development and spread of strange cells in the colon or rectum. While the specific grouping of occasions can shift from one person to another, certain hereditary transformations and cell changes assume a focal part in the turn of events and movement of the sickness.

At first, typical cells in the covering of the colon or rectum might procure hereditary changes that lead to the development of little, noncancerous developments called polyps. Over the long run, certain hereditary and epigenetic changes can happen inside these polyps, making them dysplastic or precancerous. Assuming that left untreated, these precancerous polyps can eventually form into intrusive colorectal malignant growth.

The movement of colorectal malignant growth is likewise affected by elements like aggravation, natural openings, way-of-life decisions, and hereditary inclination. Persistent irritation, as found in conditions like ulcerative colitis or Crohn's sickness, can add to the advancement of colorectal disease. Moreover, way of life factors, like a high-fat eating regimen, low fiber admission, and absence of actual work, can influence the movement of the infection.

Colorectal cancer can spread to nearby lymph nodes, invade deeper layers of the colon or rectum, and eventually metastasize to distant organs like the liver, lungs, or other parts of the body as the disease progresses. It is common for metastatic colorectal cancer to have a worse prognosis and necessitate more aggressive treatment strategies.

Understanding the science and movement of colorectal disease is instrumental in the improvement of designated treatments, customized treatment methodologies, and early location techniques. Research endeavors zeroed in on disentangling the atomic systems driving the movement of colorectal malignant growth keep on revealing new experiences into the sickness, prompting progress in the accuracy of medication and imaginative therapy modalities.

By revealing insight into the science and movement of colorectal malignant growth, medical services experts can pursue early discovery, risk appraisal, and customized mediations that expect to further develop results and personal satisfaction for people impacted by this sickness. Also, public mindfulness and schooling about the elements adding to the movement of colorectal malignant growth can advance proactive measures for avoidance and early mediation.

Chapter 4: Diagnosis and Screening Strategies

Colorectal malignant growth is ordinarily analyzed through a mix of clinical history, actual assessment, and screening tests. Coming up next are some normal finding and evaluating procedures for colorectal malignant growth:

1. Clinical history and actual assessment: A patient's clinical history, including side effects and family background of colorectal malignant growth, is thought about. An actual assessment, including a computerized rectal test, may likewise be performed.

2. Waste mysterious blood test (FOBT): This test recognizes the presence of blood in the stool, which can be an early sign of colorectal disease or other gastrointestinal issues. A basic and painless test can be performed at home.

3. Colonoscopy: A colonoscopy involves inserting a long, flexible tube into the colon with a camera at the end to directly observe the rectum and colon lining. This takes into consideration the discovery of polyps, unusual developments, or different indications of colorectal malignant growth. If irregularities are found, a biopsy might be taken for additional assessment.

4. Adaptable sigmoidoscopy: Like a colonoscopy, this strategy likewise utilizes an adaptable cylinder with a camera to inspect the lower part of the colon and rectum. In any case, it doesn't venture as far into the colon as a colonoscopy.

5. CT colonography (virtual colonoscopy): Using a CT scanner, this non-invasive imaging procedure produces precise images of the rectum and colon. For some patients, it is an alternative to a conventional colonoscopy.

6. Stool DNA test: Stool DNA markers that are linked to colorectal cancer are looked for by this test. It could be utilized as an option to or related to other screening tests.

7. Blood tests: The levels of certain substances in the blood that can indicate the presence of colorectal cancer can be monitored using blood tests like the carcinoembryonic antigen (CEA) test.

The American Disease Society suggests standard colorectal malignant growth screenings for people at normal gamble beginning at age 45. However, a person's risk factors, family history, and preferences may differ from one screening strategy to the next. To figure out which screening option is best for each person, it's important to talk about it with a doctor.

Discussing different screening methods

There are a few screening strategies accessible for colorectal disease, each with its advantages and contemplations. Two significant evaluating strategies for colorectal malignant growth are colonoscopies and hereditary testing.

1. Colonoscopy:

The most effective method for detecting colorectal cancer is a colonoscopy. During this technique, a long, adaptable cylinder with a camera toward the end is embedded into the colon to inspect the whole length of the colon and rectum.

- Colonoscopies can recognize and eliminate precancerous polyps, as well as distinguish beginning phase colorectal disease. This can assist with forestalling colorectal malignant growth by eliminating polyps before they become harmful.

- While colonoscopies are exceptionally successful, they are an intrusive strategy that requires gut readiness and sedation. A few people may likewise encounter uneasiness and minor dangers like draining or inside holes.

2. Hereditary Testing:

- Hereditary testing for colorectal disease includes dissecting an individual's hereditary cosmetics to recognize changes or modifications in unambiguous qualities that are related to an expanded gamble of creating colorectal malignant growth. One of the most notable hereditary circumstances related to colorectal disease is the Lynch condition.

- Individuals with a potential hereditary predisposition to colorectal cancer can be identified through genetic testing, prompting them to undergo more frequent or specialized screening as well as cascade testing for family members.

- While hereditary testing gives significant data, taking into account the mental and close-to-home ramifications of finding out about an expanded gamble of creating colorectal cancer is fundamental. Furthermore, the expense and accessibility of hereditary testing might be boundaries for certain people.

Other Screening Strategies:

Notwithstanding colonoscopy and hereditary testing, there are different other evaluating strategies for colorectal malignant growth, including:

- Waste Mysterious Blood Test (FOBT) and Waste Immunochemical Test (FIT): These painless tests identify blood in the stool, which might show the presence of colorectal disease or polyps.

- CT Colonography (Virtual Colonoscopy): This imaging test utilizes processed tomography (CT) to make itemized pictures of the colon and rectum. It is a harmless option in contrast to customary colonoscopy.

- Sigmoidoscopy with Flexibility: Like a colonoscopy, this method looks at the lower part of the colon and rectum utilizing an adaptable cylinder with a camera. Be that as it may, it doesn't venture as far into the colon as a colonoscopy.

People genuinely must talk about their screening choices with their medical services suppliers to decide the most suitable strategy given their age, risk variables, and individual inclinations. Normal screenings are vital for early location and counteraction of colorectal disease.

Exploring the benefits of early detection and identifying high-risk individuals

The advantages of early discovery of colorectal disease are critical, and recognizing high-risk people is fundamental for executing fitting screening and preventive systems.

Advantages of early discovery of colorectal cancer:

1. Further developed Treatment Results: Early recognition of colorectal disease can prompt better treatment choices and further developed endurance rates. At the point when colorectal malignant growth is analyzed at the beginning phase before it has spread, it is many times more treatable with a higher opportunity of fruitful results.

2. Prevention: Screening tests, for example, colonoscopies can distinguish and eliminate precancerous polyps before they progress to become harmful. This forestalls the advancement of colorectal disease and diminishes the requirement for additional obtrusive medicines.

3. Less Obtrusive Medicines: Beginning phase colorectal disease might be treated with less intrusive surgeries, decreasing the effect on the patient's satisfaction and the requirement for broad treatment.

4. Decreased Mortality: Distinguishing and treating colorectal malignant growth at a beginning phase can altogether decrease the gamble of mortality related to the illness.

Recognizing high-risk people:

1. Family Ancestry: Having a first-degree relative (parent, kin, or kid) with colorectal malignant growth or certain acquired disorders, for example,

Lynch's condition can essentially build a singular gamble of fostering the sickness.

2. Hereditary Inclination: Certain hereditary changes, like transformations in the APC, MLH1, MSH2, MSH6, PMS2, and EPCAM qualities, are related to an expanded gamble of colorectal disease. Hereditary testing can assist in recognizing people with these changes and evaluate their gamble.

3. Personal History of Polyps or Colorectal Cancer: People who have had a past conclusion of colorectal malignant growth or particular kinds of polyps are at an expanded gamble of fostering the illness once more, requiring nearer checking and reconnaissance.

4. Fiery Inside Sickness: Colorectal cancer is more likely to occur in people who have Crohn's disease or ulcerative colitis, especially if the condition affects a large portion of the colon and has been present for a long time.

By recognizing people with these high-risk factors, medical care suppliers can suggest customized screening systems and reconnaissance plans custom-made to every individual's profile. This might incorporate starting screening at a previous age, more successive screening stretches, and the utilization of further developed screening techniques like colonoscopies and hereditary testing. Early location and customized observation can assume an essential part in diminishing the occurrence and mortality of colorectal malignant growth in high-risk people.

Chapter 5: Battling against Colorectal Cancer

Colorectal malignant growth is an unavoidable and possibly dangerous infection that influences the colon or rectum. Combating against this sort of disease requires a complete methodology including clinical treatment, consistent encouragement, and way of life changes.

As far as clinical therapy, there are different choices accessible depending upon the stage and seriousness of the malignant growth. These could be radiation therapy to target the affected area, chemotherapy to kill cancer cells, surgery to remove the tumor, or a combination of these treatments. Individuals who have been diagnosed with colorectal cancer must collaborate closely with their healthcare team to choose the best course of action.

Aside from clinical intercessions, daily reassurance is significant while engaging against colorectal malignant growth. It's not unexpected to encounter dread, uneasiness, and stress during such a difficult time. Looking for direction from advisors, joining support gatherings, or conversing with loved ones can assist with lightening a portion of these close-to-home weights. Keep in mind that you're in good company in this battle.

Moreover, embracing a sound way of life can supplement clinical medicines and add to generally speaking prosperity. A well-balanced diet that includes lean proteins, whole grains, fruits, and vegetables can provide essential nutrients and lower the likelihood of recurrence. Standard activity keeps up with actual wellness and further develops energy levels, while likewise helping emotional well-being.

Early recognition must play a huge part in fruitful treatment results. Customary screenings, for example, colonoscopies and waste mysterious blood tests, are suggested, particularly for people over the age of 50 or those with a family background of colorectal disease. Distinguishing disease at a beginning phase expands the possibilities of successful treatment and long-haul endurance.

Ultimately, remaining positive and keeping a confident viewpoint can have a critical effect on the fight against colorectal disease. Encircling oneself with strong people, participating in exercises that give pleasure, and putting forth practical objectives can assist with cultivating versatility all through the excursion.

Keep in mind, that each individual's involvement in engaging colorectal disease is novel. Counseling medical services experts for customized exhortation and guidance is fundamental. One can increase their chances of overcoming colorectal cancer and leading a fulfilling life by taking a proactive approach, cultivating emotional well-being, adopting a healthy lifestyle, and seeking appropriate medical treatment.

Engaging against colorectal malignant growth frequently includes a complete methodology that incorporates a mix of medicines like a medical procedure, chemotherapy, and immunotherapy. Here are a few features of the most recent therapy choices for colorectal disease:

1. Surgery:

Medical procedure is many times the underlying therapy for colorectal malignant growth and is utilized to eliminate carcinogenic cancers and any close by impacted tissue. Progresses in careful methods, like negligibly obtrusive systems and mechanical helped a medical procedure, have prompted diminished recuperation times, less post-usable torment, and further developed results for patients.

The use of laparoscopic and robotic procedures makes it possible to remove tumors through smaller incisions, which results in shorter hospital stays and quicker recovery. In situations where the disease has metastasized to the liver, careful methods, for example, liver resection or radiofrequency removal might be used to eliminate or obliterate the malignant sores.

2. Chemotherapy:

Chemotherapy is a foundational therapy that utilizations medications to kill disease cells or stop their development. The utilization of targeted therapies, which target specific abnormalities within cancer cells, is one of the most recent advancements in colorectal cancer chemotherapy. For instance, tranquilizers that focus on the epidermal development factor receptor (EGFR) or vascular endothelial development factor (VEGF) have shown adequacy in cutting-edge colorectal disease by restricting the development of growths and dragging out endurance.

3. Immunotherapy:

Immunotherapy has arisen as a promising therapy choice for colorectal malignant growth. It works by helping the body's safe framework to perceive and go after disease cells. Resistant designated spot inhibitors, for example, pembrolizumab and nivolumab, have shown viability in patients with microsatellite unsteadiness high (MSI-H) or befuddle fix lacking (dMMR) growths, prompting FDA endorsement for use in metastatic colorectal disease.

Blend treatments that incorporate immunotherapy and other designated therapies are likewise being investigated as a method for upgrading the safe reaction and further developing results in colorectal disease patients.

Precision medicine approaches are being used to identify specific genetic alterations in tumors, allowing for the use of personalized therapies that target the particular molecular characteristics of an individual's cancer in addition to these traditional treatment options.

It's critical to take note that the decision of therapy relies upon different factors like the phase of the malignant growth, the patient's general well-being, and the particular atomic attributes of the cancer. Multidisciplinary care including oncologists, specialists, hereditary advisors, and different experts is urgent in deciding the best treatment plan customized to every patient's necessities.

Overall, the most recent advancements in colorectal cancer treatment offer patients fighting this disease hope for better outcomes and improved quality of life.

Importance of personalized treatment plans

When fighting colorectal cancer, it's critical to stress the significance of individualized treatment plans that are tailored to each patient's unique circumstances. Customized therapy considers the special qualities of an individual's malignant growth, as well as their general well-being, hereditary cosmetics, and individual inclinations. This approach can essentially influence treatment adequacy and the personal satisfaction of patients. The following are a few vital parts of customized therapy plans for colorectal malignant growth:

1. Genetic Testing:

Understanding the hereditary profile of the disease can direct treatment choices. The selection of targeted therapies, immunotherapies, and clinical trial opportunities may be influenced by specific mutations or biomarkers that can be found through genetic testing. For example, distinguishing microsatellite insecurity (MSI) or bungle fix inadequacy (dMMR) can assist with deciding if safe designated spot inhibitors are proper.

2. Tumor Molecular Profiling:

The tumor's unique biological characteristics can be uncovered through advanced molecular profiling, which has the potential to identify genetic alterations that could be targeted. This permits oncologists to choose treatments that are probably going to be compelling for the singular's disease while limiting superfluous openness to medicines with restricted benefits.

3. Stage and Location of the Cancer:

The precise stage and location of colorectal cancer are crucial to the planning of treatment. Customized therapy plans consider whether the malignant growth has spread, the size and area of the cancer, and whether it influences close by organs or lymph hubs.

4. Treatment Preferences and Goals:

A personalized treatment plan must take into account the treatment preferences, lifestyle, and personal objectives of the patient. A few patients might focus on limiting treatment secondary effects and saving personal satisfaction, while others might want more forceful treatment to boost endurance results.

5. Multidisciplinary Care:

A customized approach includes joint effort among a multidisciplinary group of subject matter experts, including clinical oncologists, careful oncologists, radiation oncologists, hereditary guides, and other medical services experts. This group cooperates to foster individualized treatment procedures and gives exhaustive consideration that tends to all parts of the patient's prosperity.

6. Supportive Care:

Customized treatment designs likewise envelop strong consideration measures to oversee side effects, work on personal satisfaction, and address the mental and profound requirements of the patient. This might include tormenting the board, wholesome help, directing, and other steady administrations.

The idea of customized medication in colorectal malignant growth treatment highlights the shift towards accuracy and custom-made treatments. By perceiving the interesting elements of every patient's malignant growth, customized treatment plans amplify the probability of treatment accomplishment while limiting superfluous treatment-related harmfulness.

In the end, the goal of personalized treatment plans is to make it easier for patients to actively participate in their care decisions, improve the patient experience, and improve patient outcomes. This approach recognizes the intricacies of colorectal disease and plans to give designated, powerful, and patient-focused care.

Chapter 6: Embracing a Lifestyle Shield

Embracing a way of life safeguard is a fundamental technique in forestalling colorectal disease. A way-of-life safeguard includes embracing solid propensities, including a reasonable eating routine, standard activity, and other positive way-of-life decisions that can essentially decrease the gamble of creating colorectal malignant growth. By tending to the job of diet, workout, and sound propensities, people can proactively pursue decreasing their gamble of this sickness. The following are a few vital parts of a way of life safeguard:

1. Diet:

Eating an eating regimen wealthy in organic products, vegetables, entire grains, and incline proteins can have a defensive impact against colorectal malignant growth. Consuming various brilliant foods grown from the ground gives fundamental supplements, fiber, and cancer prevention agents, which might assist with lessening aggravation and forestall harm to colon cells. Furthermore, restricting the utilization of handled meats and red meats, which have been connected to an expanded gamble of colorectal disease, is suggested.

2. Active work:

Standard actual work is related to a diminished gamble of colorectal disease. Taking part in moderate to lively activity, like energetic strolling, running, swimming, or cycling, for somewhere around 150 minutes the week can give critical defensive advantages. Practice adds to generally speaking well-being by advancing the sound weight of the executives, working on stomach-related capability, and decreasing irritation.

3. Controlling your weight:

To lower one's risk of developing colorectal cancer, it is essential to maintain a healthy weight. Being overweight or fat is a critical gamble element, and an overabundance of muscle-to-fat ratio, especially around the waistline, is related to an improved probability of creating colorectal malignant growth. Keeping a close eye on one's weight and working to reach and maintain a healthy weight range can help prevent disease.

4. Restricting Liquor and Tobacco Use:

The utilization of liquor and tobacco has been connected to an expanded gamble of colorectal malignant growth. Restricting or staying away from liquor utilization and forgoing smoking can decrease the gamble of fostering this type of disease and offer more extensive medical advantages.

5. Screening and Early Recognition:

Sticking to routine evaluating suggestions for colorectal malignant growth, especially for people at normal gamble and those with family ancestry, is essential. Normal screenings can prompt early location and give the open door to opportune intercession and treatment.

6. Choices for a Healthy Lifestyle:

Taking on another solid way of life rehearses, for example, getting adequate rest, overseeing pressure, and getting customary preventive medical care, adds to general prosperity and can by implication add to colorectal disease avoidance.

Individuals can help reduce their risk of colorectal cancer by adopting a lifestyle that includes a healthy diet, regular exercise, and positive habits. Beyond colorectal cancer prevention, proactive efforts to maintain a healthy lifestyle support overall health and well-being. Moreover, consolidating these practices right off the bat in life can lay out an establishment for long-haul colorectal malignant growth counteraction and in general well-being advancement.

Practical tips for reducing risk factors and maintaining overall well-being

Colorectal disease is a common type of malignant growth that influences the colon or rectum. While specific gamble factors for colorectal diseases, like age and family ancestry, can't be controlled, embracing a way of life safeguard can fundamentally diminish the gamble and advance generally speaking prosperity. This article plans to give down-to-earth tips for diminishing gambling factors and keeping a solid way of life to forestall colorectal malignant growth.

1. Eat a Reasonable Eating regimen:

An eating regimen rich in natural products, vegetables, entire grains, and incline proteins can assist with decreasing the gamble of colorectal malignant growth. Incorporate high-fiber food sources like beans, lentils, and entire grains in your dinners. Red and processed meats have been linked to an increased risk, so cut them out. Choose better cooking strategies like barbecuing, baking, or steaming as opposed to searing.

2. Remain Truly Dynamic:

Customary actual work is vital in diminishing the gamble of colorectal malignant growth. Go for the gold 150 minutes of moderate-power high-impact practice or 75 minutes of fiery activity each week. Participate in exercises you appreciate, like lively strolling, cycling, swimming, or moving. Active work lessens the gamble of disease as well as works on generally speaking prosperity.

3. Keep a Solid Weight:

Colorectal cancer risk has been linked to obesity and excess body weight. Endeavor to keep a sound load through a mix of a decent eating regimen and ordinary activity. Counsel medical services proficient or an enrolled dietitian for customized direction on weight the board.

4. Limit Liquor Utilization:

Consumption of excessive alcohol has been linked to an increased risk of colorectal cancer. Be careful not to consume too much alcoholic beverages. The American Malignant Growth Society prescribes restricting liquor admission to something like two beverages each day for men and one beverage for ladies.

5. Stop Smoking:

Smoking is a critical gamble factor for different sorts of diseases, including colorectal malignant growth. Stopping smoking lessens the gamble of malignant growth as well as works on general well-being. Look for help from medical care experts, support gatherings, or smoking discontinuance projects to assist you with stopping smoking effectively.

6. Monitor frequently:

Standard evaluation for colorectal malignant growth is fundamental for early recognition and counteraction. Adhere to the suggested screening rules in light of your age and hazard factors. Screening procedures such as colonoscopies, fecal occult blood tests, and others can assist in the identification of precancerous polyps or early-stage cancer, thereby increasing the likelihood of successful treatment.

7. Importance of personalized treatment plans

Stress can hurt one's overall health and raise the risk of colorectal cancer. Engaging in hobbies, practicing relaxation techniques, or seeking support from loved ones are all healthy ways to manage stress. Consider integrating pressure-lessening exercises like yoga, reflection, or care into your everyday daily schedule.

Embracing a way of life safeguard for colorectal disease includes pursuing cognizant decisions to lessen risk factors and keep up with general prosperity. By embracing a reasonable eating regimen, remaining genuinely dynamic, keeping a solid weight, restricting liquor utilization, stopping smoking, going through normal screenings, and overseeing pressure, you can essentially decrease the gamble of colorectal disease. Keep in mind that counteraction is vital, and little way of life changes can have a major effect on your wellbeing. Begin carrying out these commonsense tips today and assume command over your prosperity.

Chapter 7: Turning the Tables: Survivor Stories

Colorectal malignant growth is a difficult illness that influences a large number of individuals around the world. In any case, amid the challenges, there are endless moving accounts of people who have dealt with this conclusion directly and arose triumphant. These accounts act as an encouraging sign, helping us to remember the flexibility and strength of the human soul. In this article, we will share a couple of surprising accounts of people who have beaten colorectal disease, filling in as a motivation to others confronting comparative fights.

1. Sarah's Story:
Sarah was determined to have colorectal disease very early in life, which came as a shock to her and her friends and family. Regardless of the close-to-home and actual difficulties, Sarah moved toward her treatment with

unflinching assurance. She went through a medical procedure, trailed by chemotherapy and radiation. All through her excursion, she kept an uplifting perspective, encircled herself with a solid emotionally supportive network, and took part in exercises that gave her pleasure. Today, Sarah is malignant growth-free and has turned into a backer for bringing issues to light about colorectal disease in youthful grown-ups.

2. John's Journey:

John, a moderately aged man, was determined to have progressed stage colorectal disease. The forecast was dreary, however John would not surrender. He searched out the best clinical specialists, investigated elective treatment choices, and made a huge way of life changes. John likewise joined help gatherings, where he found comfort and consolation from others confronting comparable difficulties. Through his assurance and the help of his friends and family, John resisted the chances and is currently carrying on with a satisfying life, malignant growth-free.

3. Emily's Victory:

Emily's excursion with colorectal malignant growth was a long and challenging one. She got through different medical procedures, chemotherapy, and radiation, all while adjusting her obligations as a mother and spouse. Despite the physical and close-to-home cost, Emily never lost trust. She tracked down comfort in journaling, offering her viewpoints and feelings all through her treatment. Emily's steadfast soul and strength assisted her with defeating disease as well as enlivened others locally to remain solid notwithstanding difficulty.

4. Mark's Miracle:

Mark's story is one of trust and steadiness. Determined to have late-stage colorectal malignant growth, Imprint was given a hopeless guess. Notwithstanding, he would not acknowledge it as his destiny. Mark searched out clinical preliminaries and, not entirely set in stone to track down an answer. His immovable assurance paid off when he turned into a piece of a noteworthy treatment that prompted reduction. Imprint's story fills in as a demonstration of the force of never surrendering, even despite outlandish chances.

The tales of people who have won over colorectal disease are a demonstration of the dauntless human soul. These rousing people confronted their conclusion with fortitude, flexibility, and a faithful assurance to survive. Their accounts advise us that there is trust, even in the haziest of times. By sharing their encounters, they rouse others to have faith in their solidarity and battle against this illness. These momentous people act as encouraging signs, showing us that with the right attitude, backing, and clinical consideration, it is feasible to conquer colorectal malignant growth and arise more grounded on the opposite side.

Encouraging expectation and flexibility despite colorectal disease includes recognizing the difficulties while stressing positive survival strategies. Empowering a steady organization of companions, family, and medical care experts is vital. Giving solid data about treatment choices and advances can enable people to confront the excursion with more noteworthy flexibility. Furthermore, advancing a sound way of life, including legitimate sustenance and exercise, adds to generally speaking prosperity. Coordinating psychological well-being backing and directing assists people with exploring the profound parts of their excursion, encouraging a feeling of trust and strength despite misfortune.

How has advancement in medical treatment improved outcomes for patients?

Headways in clinical therapy for colorectal malignant growth have further developed results for patients. One huge headway is the advancement of designated treatments that can explicitly go after malignant growth cells, limiting harm to sound tissues. These designated treatments, like monoclonal antibodies and safe designated spot inhibitors, have shown promising outcomes in further developing endurance rates.

The development of surgical methods has also made it possible for less invasive and more precise procedures. This lessens the gamble of complexities and further develops recuperation time for patients. Mechanical medical procedure is one such method that has acquired fame as of late.

Moreover, there have been progressions in chemotherapy choices, with the improvement of new medications and treatment regimens. These progressions have expanded the viability of chemotherapy as well as diminished its secondary effects, bringing about superior personal satisfaction for patients going through treatment.

Generally, these headways in clinical therapy have prompted superior results for colorectal disease patients, including higher endurance rates and better personal satisfaction during and after treatment. Nonetheless, it's memorable's critical that each case is special, and customized exhortation from medical care experts is fundamental for settling on informed therapy choices.

To educate the general public about colorectal cancer, its symptoms, and the resources available to patients, caregivers, and their families, it is essential to promote support and awareness of the disease. By expanding mindfulness, we can empower early recognition and brief clinical consideration, at last further developing results for those impacted by colorectal malignant growth.

One successful approach to spreading mindfulness is through instructive missions. These missions can use different mediums like TV, radio, virtual entertainment, and print materials to contact a wide crowd. By giving exact and exceptional data about colorectal disease, its gamble variables, side effects, and screening strategies, these missions can assist people with grasping the significance of early identification and safeguard measures.

Moreover, support gatherings and online networks assume an urgent part in offering profound and functional help to those impacted by colorectal disease. Support gatherings can unite patients, survivors, guardians, and their families, permitting them to share their encounters, difficulties, and ways of dealing with stress. These gatherings give a place of refuge to people to communicate their sentiments, look for counsel, and find comfort in realizing they are in good company on their excursion.

Online people groups likewise offer a significant stage for sharing data, assets, and backing. Through gatherings, discussion boards, and web-based entertainment gatherings, people can interface with other people who have comparable encounters and get an abundance of information and direction. Online people groups can likewise assist with bringing issues to light about colorectal malignant growth by sharing individual stories, raising money endeavors, and pertinent news and exploration discoveries.

Furthermore, medical services experts and associations can use computer-based intelligence stages such as myself to scatter exact and forward-thinking data about colorectal disease. Through intelligent discussions, I can give direction on normal inquiries, offer data about screening techniques, and treatment choices, and accessible encouraging groups of people. Visit man-made intelligence can act as a solid asset for people looking for data and backing, assisting with overcoming any barrier between patients, parental figures, and medical services experts.

Also, spreading mindfulness and backing for colorectal malignant growth is fundamental to further develop results and give important assets to people impacted by this illness. Through instructive missions, support gatherings, and online networks, we can provide people with information, offer basic reassurance, and associate them with the assets they need on their excursion towards better well-being.

Spreading mindfulness and backing for colorectal malignant growth includes drawing in with different drives, associations, and assets devoted to supporting patients and their families. Prominent associations like the Colorectal Disease Partnership and the American Malignant Growth Society effectively add to schooling and support. These elements offer important data on counteraction, early identification, and treatment choices.

Drives, for example, Colorectal Disease Mindfulness Month give stages to raise public cognizance. Nearby occasions, online missions, and local area outreach programs play a crucial part in scattering data.

Assets accessible for patients and families incorporate help hotlines, directing administrations, and instructive materials presented by associations like Battle Colorectal Disease. These assets plan to offer profound help, self-direction, and cutting-edge data all through the disease venture.

By encouraging joint efforts between these drives, associations, and assets, we can aggregately reinforce the battle against colorectal malignant growth and further develop the general prosperity of those impacted by this sickness.

Pushing for expanded public mindfulness and early location crusades in colorectal malignant growth is basic to lessen the weight of this sickness. It is essential to collaborate with healthcare professionals, community leaders, and advocacy groups to design and carry out effective awareness campaigns.

Instructive missions ought to accentuate the significance of customary screenings, perceiving side effects, and understanding gambling factors. Using different media channels, including online entertainment, television, and print, can contact assorted crowds successfully.

Drawing in people of note and powerhouses to share individual stories or take part in mindfulness occasions can improve crusade permeability. Additionally, expanding your reach is made possible by collaborating with healthcare providers to provide easy-to-access screening programs, particularly in underserved communities.

By supporting expanded mindfulness and early recognition, we can enable people to go to proactive lengths, eventually further developing colorectal disease results through ideal conclusion and intercession.

To guarantee that people who have colorectal cancer receive the information, resources, and emotional support they require, it is essential to raise awareness of the disease and offer assistance to those who have it. There are a few drives, associations, and assets accessible that expect to address these necessities and engage patients and their families:

1. Mindfulness Missions: Numerous associations lead mindfulness missions to instruct the overall population about the significance of early discovery, screening, and way-of-life adjustments to forestall colorectal disease. To reach a large number of people, these campaigns make use of a variety of channels, including television, social media, and community events.

2. Non-benefit Associations: Various non-benefit associations are devoted to supporting colorectal malignant growth patients and their families. Models incorporate the Colorectal Disease Collusion, the American Malignant Growth Society, and Battle Colorectal Disease. For patients in need, these organizations provide helpful resources, support groups, educational materials, and financial assistance programs.

3. Web-Based Resources: There are a few internet-based stages that give thorough data on colorectal malignant growth, treatment choices, and steady consideration. Information such as symptom checkers, treatment guidelines, and survivorship resources can be found on trustworthy and up-to-date websites like those of the American Cancer Society (ACS) and the National Cancer Institute (NCI). M4. Patient Care Groups: Peer support assumes a fundamental part in assisting patients with adapting to the difficulties of colorectal disease. Patients and their families can find

emotional support, advice, and connections with others who have been through similar circumstances through support groups. Neighborhood emergency clinics, disease focuses, and non-benefit associations frequently work with these care groups.

4. Clinical Experts: Medical services suppliers assume a basic part in directing patients through their colorectal malignant growth venture. Doctors, medical attendants, and other medical care experts offer ability in determination, therapy, and the executive's systems. They can direct patients and their families to the right resources and services for support.

5. Screening Projects: Numerous nations have carried out coordinated screening projects to identify colorectal malignant growth at the beginning phase. These projects guarantee that people in danger get standard screening tests, for example, colonoscopies or waste mysterious blood tests. Bringing issues to light about these projects can urge more individuals to take part and possibly distinguish the sickness in its initial, more treatable stages.

By and large, spreading mindfulness about colorectal malignant growth and offering help through drives, associations, and assets is fundamental for further developing results and diminishing the effect of this illness on people and networks. By cooperating, we can have a massive effect in battling colorectal disease and working on the personal satisfaction of patients and their friends and family.

Conclusion

In conclusion, colorectal malignant growth is a serious sickness that influences a great many people around the world. All through this discussion, we have examined the significance of early recognition, normal screenings, and way-of-life changes as viable measures in forestalling and dealing with this disease. Furthermore, we have underlined the meaning of bringing issues to light, supporting drives and associations, and giving assets to battle colorectal malignant growth.

Readers need to comprehend that they can significantly impact the fight against this disease through their actions. By doing whatever it takes to teach themselves about colorectal disease, empowering customary screenings, and embracing sound way of life decisions, they can safeguard themselves and their friends and family.

Keep in mind, that early identification saves lives. Assuming you or somebody you know encounters any side effects or chance elements related to colorectal disease, go ahead and clinical consideration. Together, by uniting and pursuing a shared objective, we can beat the colorectal disease, further develop results, and improve the personal satisfaction of patients and their families. Allow us to stand joined against colorectal disease and make a move today.

Colorectal cancer represents a huge well-being challenge, yet by figuring out its stages, cultivating trust, and spreading mindfulness, we can have an effect. The significance of early identification couldn't possibly be more significant, as it altogether further develops treatment results. Drives, associations, and assets are promptly accessible to help patients and their families on this excursion.

It is more important than ever to act right now. Spread mindfulness locally, energize customary screenings, and back associations devoted to battling colorectal disease. By meeting up, we can expose the foe, advance early discovery, and eventually gain ground in diminishing the effect of colorectal disease. Allow us to join in the battle against this sickness, taking a stab at a future where colorectal malignant growth isn't simply treatable but preventable.

Promoting regular screenings, adopting a healthy lifestyle, and raising awareness are important tools in the ongoing fight against colorectal cancer. Normal screenings, like colonoscopies, assume a critical part in early identification, considering opportune mediation and further developed results.

Taking on a sound way of life, enveloping adjusted nourishment and normal activity, brings down the gamble of colorectal malignant growth as well as supports by and large prosperity. Promoting the significance of preventative measures, dispelling myths, and educating the general public about risk factors all depend on awareness campaigns.

How about we focus on our well-being by booking screenings, going with a careful way of life decisions, and effectively partaking in mindfulness crusades? Thus, we can add to the aggregate exertion in diminishing the effect of colorectal disease and cultivating a better future for all.

Colorectal cancer is a serious disease that affects the rectum. It is crucial to encourage regular screenings, as early detection can greatly increase the chances of successful treatment and improved outcomes. By promoting regular screenings, we can help individuals identify any potential issues early on and take proactive steps to address them.

In addition to screenings, promoting healthy lifestyle choices is integral in the fight against colorectal cancer. Encouraging individuals to maintain a balanced diet rich in fruits, vegetables, and whole grains can help reduce the risk of developing this disease. Regular exercise, such as brisk walking or cycling, can also lower the risk factors associated with colorectal cancer. By adopting these healthy habits, individuals can potentially reduce their chances of developing this disease.

Creating awareness about colorectal cancer is essential in empowering individuals to take charge of their health. By disseminating information about common symptoms, risk factors, and preventive measures, we can ensure that people are well-informed and proactive in seeking medical attention if needed. Education campaigns, community outreach programs, and media platforms can all play a significant role in spreading awareness and encouraging individuals to prioritize their health.

By focusing on and promoting these three key aspects - regular screenings, healthy lifestyle choices, and awareness - we can make a significant impact in the fight against colorectal cancer. Together, we have the power to improve outcomes and enhance the quality of life for patients and their families. Let us stand united and take action today to combat colorectal cancer.

www.ingramcontent.com/pod-product-compliance
Lightning Source LLC
Chambersburg PA
CBHW050748250726
48662CB00005B/2090